DANCE WITH THE SHADOW

Emotions Unveiled

Dr. Vivek S. Ph.D.

ISBN: 9798857259078

Cover design by: Art Painter
Library of Congress Control Number: 2018675309
Printed in the United States of America

To all those who dare to embark on the intimate journey of self-discovery,
To the seekers of light who courageously confront their shadows,
To the resilient hearts that find strength in vulnerability,
To the ones who understand that embracing the darkness is a step toward the light,

This book is dedicated to you.

"Dance with the Shadow" is a tribute to the complexity and beauty of the human experience. May its pages illuminate the path of self-awareness, guide you through the depths of your emotions, and empower you to waltz with your shadows in the grand ballroom of your soul.

With gratitude for your willingness to explore the uncharted territories within,

Dr. Vivek S. Ph.D.

"Embrace your shadows, for within them lies the untamed power of your true self."

— Dr. Vivek S. Ph.D., iGCBT

FOREWORD

Hello There,

I'm absolutely thrilled to introduce you to a book that's been a true labor of love for me - "Dance with the shadow: Emotions Unveiled" As you flip through these pages, you're embarking on a journey that's all about self-discovery, empowerment, and transforming the way you navigate your emotions. I'm Vivek, and I've poured my heart and expertise into every word you'll find here.

"Dance with the Shadow: Emotions Unveiled" - the title pretty much sums up what this book is all about. I'm a Mental Health Professional and a Counsellor, and my aim here is to give you the tools and insights to not only understand your emotions but to truly master them in a way that changes your life for the better.

What you'll discover within these pages is a tapestry of stories, insights, and strategies that invite you to explore the intricate landscape of your emotions. My hope is that my words will gently guide you through topics like emotional awareness, self-compassion, mindfulness, vulnerability, and the art of nurturing meaningful relationships. Each chapter is a stepping stone on a path of growth, self-reflection, and transformation.

Whether you're on a personal journey to find emotional well-being or you're a mental health professional looking to expand your knowledge, this book is designed to offer something meaningful for you. I've tried to infuse warmth and empathy into my approach, recognizing that every one of us is on a unique journey.

As you explore "Dance with the Shadow: Emotions Unveiled", let my insights become a source of comfort, inspiration, and guidance for you as you navigate the intricate landscape of your emotions. With each chapter, you're taking a step closer to truly understanding, embracing, and harnessing the power of your emotions to craft a life that's fulfilling, meaningful, and resilient.

Warm regards,

Dr. Vivek S. Ph.D.

INTRODUCTION

In today's fast-paced world, where demands and complexities seem to be ever on the rise, I'm convinced that our emotional well-being plays a crucial role in how we handle life's challenges with grace and strength. Hi, I'm Vivek, and I'm genuinely thrilled to introduce you to a book that's incredibly close to my heart - "Dance with the shadow: Emotions Unveiled"

Imagine this book as your trusted guide for navigating the intricate landscape of emotions. I've authored it, Dr. Vivek S. Ph.D. Ph.D., iGCBT, drawing upon my background as a distinguished Mental Healthcare professional and Psychosexual Counsellor. Within its pages lies a comprehensive resource that delves deep into the remarkable journey of Emotional Orgasm.

As you journey through the chapters, you'll discover a transformative approach that sheds light on how to not just comprehend but truly harness and master your emotions. My aim is to equip you with the tools needed to navigate the intricate terrain of your feelings, cultivating a sense of resilience and well-being that stands strong over time.

Each chapter is an invitation, an invitation to explore the captivating realm of emotional intelligence, vulnerability, and self-compassion. Think of it as embarking on a voyage of self-discovery and growth, where each step leads you closer to a place of inner strength and profound understanding.

It doesn't matter if you're here to enrich your emotional intelligence or to gain a deeper grasp of the world of emotions for personal growth - "Emotional Orgasm" has something to offer you. It's a beacon of light that guides you towards embracing your emotions, enhancing your well-being, and crafting a life that's genuinely fulfilling. Thank you for joining me on this exhilarating journey. Together, let's take steps towards a future marked by emotional empowerment and lasting well-being.

ACKNOWLEDGEMENTS

With deep appreciation, I thank my family and friends for their unwavering support in creating "Dance with the shadow: Emotions Unveiled" Your encouragement and patience have been priceless as I embarked on this journey.

A special gratitude to Mr. Anil Thomas, an esteemed NLP and Gestalt Facilitator, and my mentor. Your guidance shaped the ideas in this book, inspiring me to explore emotional well-being and resilience more deeply.

I am also grateful to readers and individuals who shared their stories, enriching this book with their experiences. Your openness showcases the strength of shared connections.

To the entire team behind this book – editors, designers, and publishers – thank you for your dedication and commitment to realizing this project.

Lastly, my sincere thanks to every reader joining this journey. May the insights within empower you to navigate emotions, foster resilience, and embrace lasting well-being.

With heartfelt gratitude,

Dr. Vivek S. Ph.D.

ABOUT THE AUTHOR

Dr. Vivek S. Ph.D. is a prominent mental healthcare professional hailing from India. Armed with a Ph.D. in Counselling Psychology and extensive expertise across therapeutic practices such as Neurolinguistic Programming, Cognitive Behavioral Therapy, Gestalt, and Sound Healing, Vivek embodies a multifaceted approach to enhancing mental well-being. His dedication lies in fostering emotional equilibrium and bolstering resilience, driven by a fervent desire to improve relationships and nurture emotional balance. Vivek's adeptness in therapies, psychiatry, and mental disorders equips him to guide individuals on a holistic journey towards well-being. "Dance with the Shadow: Emotions Unveiled" is a testament to his commitment to mental wellness, encapsulating a comprehensive perspective that is both enlightening and transformative.

ENDORSEMENTS

"Dr. Vivek's book, 'Dance with the Shadow: Emotions Unveiled,' is a comprehensive and insightful guide that offers readers practical tools to navigate the complex landscape of emotions. His expertise as a mental healthcare professional shines through as he delves into various therapeutic modalities and provides evidence-based strategies for enhancing emotional intelligence and well-being.

"An invaluable resource for those on a journey of self-discovery and emotional growth. Dr. Vivek's deep understanding of therapeutic techniques, combined with his compassionate guidance, makes 'Emotional Orgasm' a must-read for anyone looking to cultivate emotional resilience and lead a more fulfilling life."

Prajakta Desai, Psychologist

"An enriching journey awaits readers within the pages of 'Emotional Orgasm.' Dr. Vivek's profound insights, relatable anecdotes, and practical exercises provide a roadmap for understanding and navigating emotions. His expertise as a mental healthcare professional shines through, making this book an essential tool for anyone seeking to master their emotional landscape."

Prasshanth Jituri, Mental Health Advocate

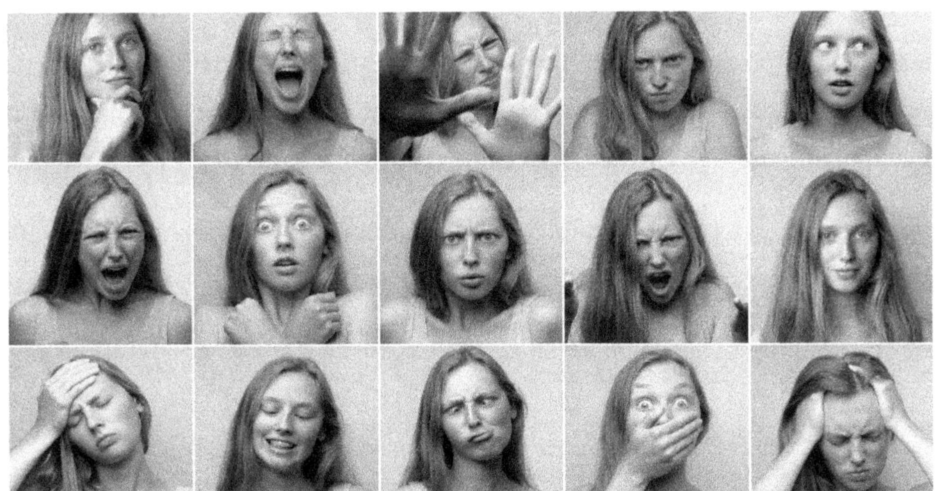

THE LANDSCAPE OF EMOTIONS

CHAPTER 1

As we begin the journey toward Emotional Orgasm, let's immerse ourselves in the captivating world of emotions. Join me, Vivek, as I guide you through the myriad feelings that color our lives, from joy and love to sorrow and anger. Within the pages of "Dance with the Shadow: Emotions Unveiled," I'm excited to share the profound concept of the "landscape of emotions."

Imagine this landscape as a canvas where each emotion paints a vivid hue on the tapestry of your inner world:

Joy: Picture yourself basking in the radiant glow of happiness, delight, and contentment. Joy often accompanies positive experiences, achievements, and meaningful connections, infusing your life with positivity and well-being.

Love: Imagine the profound embrace of intense affection and emotional attachment. Love takes on various forms, whether it's the bonds of romantic entanglement, the warmth of platonic relationships, or the transformative journey of self-love.

Sorrow: Reflect on the depths of sadness and grief that can wash over you when faced with loss, disappointment, or challenging circumstances. Sorrow is a poignant reminder of our capacity to experience and process pain.

Anger: Envision the fiery energy of anger, a powerful emotional response to perceived threats or the violation of boundaries. Anger can range from a simmering irritation to a blazing intensity, motivating us to take action or engage in meaningful communication.

Fear: Contemplate the primal instinct of fear, a deeply ingrained response to potential danger. Fear triggers the ancient "fight or flight" mechanism, serving as a vigilant guardian that keeps us safe in times of threat.

Surprise: Consider the sudden rush of surprise, an emotion that awakens your senses to novel or unexpected events. Surprise can be a delightful spark of revelation or a jolting lightning bolt of astonishment, heightening your awareness of the present moment.

Disgust: Visualize the visceral aversion of disgust, a strong reaction to something offensive or repulsive. Disgust serves as a protective shield, steering us away from potentially harmful or toxic situations.

Anticipation: Feel the eagerness and excitement that accompany the anticipation of future events and possibilities. Anticipation fuels your motivation, igniting the flames of your drive and determination.

Trust: Consider the delicate fabric of trust—a willingness to rely on and have confidence in others or in the unfolding of life's journey. Trust forms the bedrock of meaningful relationships, fostering intimacy and connection.

Sadness: Imagine the veil of sadness that may descend upon you, casting a shadow of emotional pain. Sadness invites you to delve within, encouraging introspection and reflection as you navigate life's challenges.

Happiness: Embrace the radiant state of happiness, a harmonious blend of well-being and contentment that arises from positive experiences and accomplishments.

Hope: Envision the glimmering beacon of hope, an optimistic light that illuminates the path to positive future outcomes. Hope empowers you to persevere through adversity, infusing your journey with a sense of possibility.

Each emotion carries a message—a hint about your inner world and its needs. For instance, anger might signal a need to safeguard your personal boundaries, while joy could indicate the fulfillment of a deep desire. Sadness might express a need for healing or the processing of loss, while fear might advise caution in potentially risky situations.

Understanding these emotional messages empowers you to respond consciously and effectively, making informed choices that nurture your emotional well-being and guide you toward positive outcomes. As we journey further into "Emotional Orgasm," keep these insights close, for they will be the building blocks of your emotional resilience and understanding.

The dance of emotions is a captivating symphony that weaves its melody through your thoughts, actions, and life's journey. Emotions rarely stand alone; they intertwine and converse with each other, crafting intricate patterns that paint the canvas of your emotional world. As a mental health professional and the author of "Dance with the Shadow: Emotions Unveiled," embracing this insight will equip you to guide individuals toward a profound understanding of emotional awareness and well-being.

In your journey through "Emotional Orgasm," you'll witness firsthand how emotions collaborate and converse, influencing our perceptions, decisions, and interactions. This intricate interplay is akin to a beautifully choreographed dance where each emotion takes its turn on the stage, leaving its imprint on the fabric of our experiences.

Imagine joy and sadness waltzing together, their intertwining steps creating a bittersweet melody that captures the essence of life's intricacies. Anger and fear engage in a powerful tango, each showcasing our responses to challenges and threats. Love and trust perform a harmonious duet, building the foundation of meaningful relationships.

Just as a dance troupe weaves together diverse movements to create a captivating performance, emotions unite to shape our narrative. Recognizing these connections empowers you to help others decode their emotional experiences, fostering a deeper level of self-awareness and well-being.

As you delve into the pages of this book, I invite you to explore the nuanced dialogues of emotions. Witness how they converse, amplify, or harmonize with each other. This understanding serves as a valuable tool, enabling you to guide individuals on their journey toward Emotional Orgasm.

Embrace this knowledge as a lantern that illuminates the path to emotional awareness and well-being. With every turn of the page, you're gaining insights that will enable you to offer compassionate support and guidance to those seeking a deeper connection with their emotions.

Consider the symphony of emotions:

Joy and Sadness: These emotions often dance together, creating a bittersweet symphony. Even in the midst of sadness, joy can emerge from cherished memories, offering solace and a sense of connection. Similarly, experiencing sadness can deepen the appreciation for moments of happiness, nurturing emotional resilience.

Anger and Fear: Anger and fear collaborate as guardians of your well-being. Anger may arise as a shield against perceived threats, while fear ignites the "fight or flight" response. Together, they equip you to navigate challenges, infusing you with the energy to address or avoid potential dangers.

Love and Trust: Love lays the foundation of trust in relationships. In turn, trust nurtures deeper bonds, enabling individuals to feel safe and vulnerable with each other. Love and trust intertwine, weaving a fabric of emotional security and intimacy.

Anticipation and Hope: These positive emotions join forces to ignite motivation and positive expectations. Anticipation fuels hope by envisioning favorable outcomes, while hope sustains anticipation, keeping the flame of positive possibilities alive.

Disgust and Fear: Disgust and fear collaborate to protect you from harm. Disgust acts as a deterrent from hazardous situations, while fear amplifies your avoidance response. Together, they contribute to assessing risks and ensuring self-preservation.

Surprise and Happiness: Surprise adds a touch of novelty to your life, creating openings for happiness. Positive surprises trigger feelings of joy and excitement, enriching your overall well-being.

Understanding these intricate connections empowers you to navigate emotions with finesse. For instance, recognizing that anger might stem from an underlying fear can lead to more constructive communication. Similarly, comprehending that joy can coexist with sorrow brings comfort during challenging times.

As you journey through the chapters of this book, you're embarking on an exploration of the intricate tapestry of emotional interplay. By acknowledging and delving into these nuanced connections, you'll develop emotional intelligence, bolster resilience, and cultivate a profound comprehension of your emotional experiences. This book serves as your guide to mastering the art of emotional interplay, steering you toward emotional equilibrium and lasting well-being.

Emotional intelligence (EI) acts as your compass, guiding you through the complexities of human emotions and relationships. As a mental health professional and the author of "Dance with the Shadow: Emotions Unveiled," embracing the foundations of emotional intelligence empowers you to illuminate the path toward emotional well-being for those you guide.

Self-Awareness: At the heart of emotional intelligence lies self-awareness—the profound ability to recognize and understand your own emotions. This journey involves attuning yourself to the subtleties of emotions, identifying their triggers, and decoding their impact on thoughts and behaviors. Self-awareness forms the bedrock of genuine self-understanding, laying the groundwork for improved self-regulation.

Self-Regulation: Emotional intelligence equips you with tools to adeptly manage and regulate your emotions. This entails steering clear of impulsive reactions, adapting to the ebb and flow of emotional states, and maintaining a harmonious emotional equilibrium. Through self-regulation, you acquire the ability to respond thoughtfully, nurturing healthier emotional interactions and responses.

Empathy: The gift of empathy enables you to grasp and share the emotions of others. This profound skill allows you to build deeper connections by providing support, validation, and genuine understanding. Empathy forms the cornerstone of meaningful relationships, whether personal or professional.

Social Skills: Proficiency in interpersonal skills is a hallmark of emotional intelligence. Effective communication, attentive listening, conflict resolution, and collaboration are the pillars that uphold these skills. By mastering social skills, you foster positive interactions, paving the way for enriching relationships and successful teamwork.

Motivation: Within the framework of emotional intelligence, motivation acts as the driving force channeling your emotions toward achieving your goals. Individuals with heightened emotional intelligence are often fueled by a sense of purpose, passion, and unwavering resilience. This intrinsic motivation fuels continuous growth, propelling you toward the realization of your personal and professional aspirations.

Recognizing Emotions in Others: This facet of emotional intelligence involves perceiving and accurately interpreting the emotions of others. It equips you to decipher nonverbal cues, facial expressions, and body language, enhancing your ability to connect and communicate effectively.

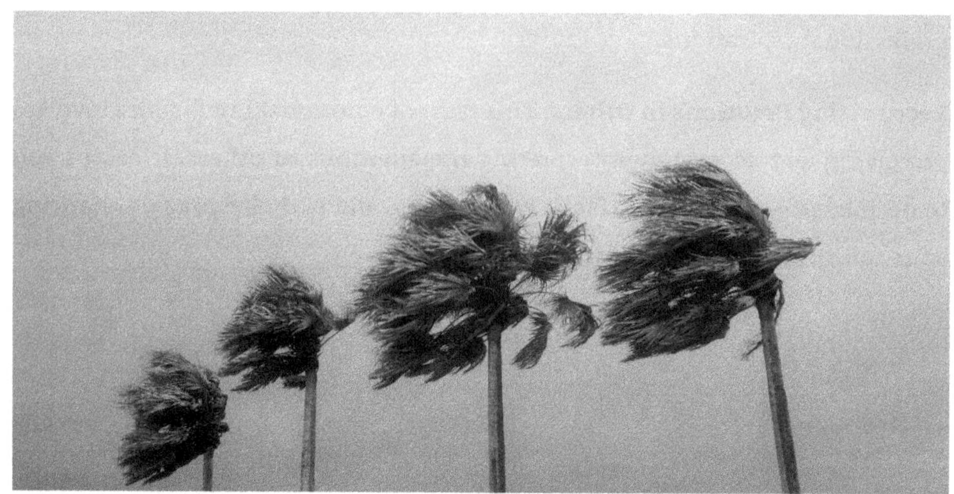

NAVIGATING LIFE's CHALLENGES
CHAPTER 2

Life is an intricate tapestry woven with challenges that can sometimes disrupt our emotional balance. In this chapter, I'm excited to share evidence-based strategies to help you navigate stress, anxiety, and adversity. Through practical exercises and real-life case studies, you'll learn how to cultivate emotional resilience when facing life's trials. My compassionate approach empowers you to see challenges as opportunities for growth, transforming emotional struggles into stepping stones toward greater well-being.

This chapter is your compass, guiding you with evidence-based strategies to navigate the turbulent waters of stress, anxiety, and adversity.

Life's journey is filled with twists and turns, presenting challenges that can shake the very core of our emotional equilibrium. At times, these challenges arrive like unexpected storms, disrupting the calm waters within us. In this chapter, we delve into the complexities of how life's trials can unsettle our emotional harmony, leaving us vulnerable to stress, anxiety, and adversity.

Drawing upon extensive research and practical expertise, I offer you evidence-based strategies that can serve as guiding lights during moments of turbulence. These strategies, grounded in scientific understanding, are far from mere speculation; they have been meticulously crafted to provide you with the tools necessary to navigate through rough seas.

The path toward emotional resilience is paved with practical exercises, offering you firsthand experience with these strategies. Through these exercises, you'll uncover the transformative potential of mindfulness, cognitive reframing, and relaxation techniques. Each exercise represents a step toward cultivating emotional resilience, equipping you to stand strong amidst life's challenges.

Moreover, real-life case studies illuminate this path, sharing the stories of individuals who have faced similar challenges. These stories, drawn from the fabric of real experiences, offer insights into how these strategies can be applied in everyday situations. Through these narratives, you'll witness the metamorphosis of emotional struggles into opportunities for enhanced well-being.

At the heart of this chapter lies a deep realization: challenges, while formidable, carry the seeds of growth within them. With compassion as our guide, I invite you to view challenges as catalysts for personal and emotional development. By embracing these challenges, along with the discomfort they bring, you set forth on a journey of profound transformation—a journey that ultimately leads to an elevated state of well-being.

Case Study 1: Sarah's Anxiety Battle

Background: Sarah, a 30-year-old marketing professional, started experiencing severe anxiety after a major client presentation went awry. She constantly worried about making mistakes and being judged by others, both at work and in her personal life.

Emotional Imbalance: Sarah's anxiety affected her sleep, appetite, and overall well-being. She withdrew from social activities and struggled to focus on her tasks at work.

Challenges: The emotional imbalance made it difficult for Sarah to perform well at her job and maintain healthy relationships. Her self-esteem plummeted, and she felt isolated.

Strategies: Sarah sought therapy and learned coping techniques such as deep breathing, mindfulness, and cognitive reframing. She also gradually exposed herself to anxiety-inducing situations to desensitize herself.

Outcome: Over time, Sarah's anxiety lessened. She gained better control over her thoughts and emotions. She continued therapy to strengthen her emotional resilience and eventually returned to a healthier work-life balance.

Case Study 2: Raj's Depression Journey

Background: Raj, a 25-year-old student, experienced a series of personal setbacks, including a breakup and academic pressures. He began feeling overwhelmed, sad, and disconnected from his passions.

Emotional Imbalance: Raj's depression led to a lack of energy, difficulty concentrating, and loss of interest in activities he once enjoyed. He started isolating himself from friends and family.

Challenges: Raj's emotional imbalance hindered his academic performance and hindered his ability to connect with others, worsening his feelings of isolation.

Strategies: Raj sought professional help and engaged in talk therapy. He also incorporated physical exercise, journaling, and reconnecting with hobbies he used to love.

Outcome: Gradually, Raj's mood improved. Through therapy, he gained insight into his negative thought patterns and learned healthier ways to cope. He rebuilt his social connections and completed his studies successfully.

Case Study 3: Priya's Grief and Resilience

Background: Priya, a 40-year-old mother of two, lost her husband in a tragic accident. She was overwhelmed by grief, experiencing intense sadness and struggling to find a sense of purpose.

Emotional Imbalance: Priya's grief manifested as a deep emotional pain that affected her ability to function. She often felt guilty for moments of joy and had difficulty adjusting to her new role as a single parent.

Challenges: Managing her own grief while supporting her children was a significant challenge. Priya's emotional imbalance also strained her relationship with her kids.

Strategies: Priya joined a grief support group, which provided a safe space to express her feelings. She also engaged in therapy to learn how to navigate her complex emotions and developed a routine that included self-care activities.

Outcome: Over time, Priya's emotional pain lessened, and she found healthier ways to honor her husband's memory. Through therapy, she gained tools to support her children's grief process and rebuilt a more meaningful life for her family.

Case Study 4: Aman's Social Anxiety

Background: Aman, a 28-year-old software engineer, struggled with social anxiety since his teenage years. He found it extremely challenging to initiate and maintain conversations, even with close friends and family.

Emotional Imbalance: Aman's social anxiety led to feelings of intense self-consciousness, fear of judgment, and avoidance of social situations. This affected his ability to form meaningful relationships and advance in his career.

Challenges: His emotional imbalance hindered his professional growth, as he avoided team meetings and networking events. It also impacted his self-esteem, contributing to a sense of isolation.

Strategies: Aman began cognitive-behavioral therapy (CBT), where he learned to challenge negative thoughts and beliefs about himself. He gradually exposed himself to social situations, starting with small gatherings and progressing to larger events.

Outcome: With consistent effort and therapy, Aman's social anxiety diminished. He gained confidence in his social interactions and started participating more actively in work-related activities. He developed new friendships and improved his overall quality of life.

Case Study 5: Maya's Post-Traumatic Growth

Background: Maya, a 35-year-old teacher, survived a serious car accident that left her with physical injuries and emotional trauma. She experienced recurring nightmares, flashbacks, and anxiety related to the accident.

Emotional Imbalance: Maya's emotional imbalance from the trauma affected her ability to feel safe, disrupted her sleep, and caused her to withdraw from her hobbies and social activities.

Challenges: The emotional turmoil made it difficult for Maya to engage fully in her work and connect with her students. She struggled to process her emotions and find a sense of meaning in the aftermath of the accident.

Strategies: Maya sought therapy to address her trauma and develop coping skills. She explored mindfulness meditation, journaling, and creative expression as outlets for her emotions.

Outcome: Through therapy, Maya worked through her trauma and gradually experienced post-traumatic growth. She gained a new perspective on life, developed greater resilience, and deepened her relationships with loved ones. Maya also became an advocate for mental health awareness and shared her journey to inspire others.

Within these case studies, you'll encounter vivid portrayals of the intricate nature of emotional imbalances. These stories highlight the spectrum of challenges that arise and the diverse strategies individuals employ to navigate their difficulties, ultimately achieving personal growth.

Life's journey is a mosaic of moments—some joyous, others challenging—each contributing to our tapestry of experience. Through twists and turns, highs and lows, we encounter unexpected trials that test our resilience and emotional equilibrium. While our natural inclination might be to seek comfort and stability, it's often in the face of these very challenges that we find the fertile ground for profound personal growth and heightened well-being.

Adopting the perspective of challenges as opportunities for growth is akin to opening a door to transformation. By reframing our mindset, we can begin to view emotional struggles not as obstacles, but as stepping stones toward a more resilient and fulfilling life. As we navigate these challenges, we unveil our capacity to evolve, learn, and thrive.

The Nature of Challenges: Catalysts for Growth

Life unfolds as a dynamic journey, marked by a diverse array of challenges that come in various forms, each bearing its own distinct shape and influence. These challenges traverse a broad spectrum, spanning from the intricacies of personal relationships and the pursuit of professional goals to the broader landscapes of societal complexities. What sets a challenge apart from a mere obstacle is its inherent ability to serve as a powerful catalyst, igniting the flames of growth and sparking transformation.

Emotional Struggles: The Underlying Landscape

Emotional battles frequently entwine themselves with the challenges we face, creating intricate layers of complexity within our journey. Emotions such as anxiety, grief, and self-doubt can cast a shadow over these challenges, seemingly magnifying their weight and rendering them formidable. However, it's crucial to understand that these emotions are not markers of surrender; rather, they signify our inherent ability to experience, introspect, and, in the end, to transform.

Beyond Roadblocks: Embracing Transformation

Inclinations often lead us to perceive challenges as obstacles, barricading our path and obstructing progress. Yet, this limited perspective belies the true potential they hold for our growth. By shifting our vantage point, we unveil a different truth: challenges are not mere roadblocks but potent catalysts that set ablaze the fires of change within us. They beckon us to confront our boundaries, to scrutinize our preconceptions, and to flexibly adjust to novel conditions. In this journey, we unlock the dormant power within us—the power to transform.

The Seeds of Resilience: Nurturing Growth

Much like a seed requires adversity to burgeon into a robust and tenacious plant, our own personal growth thrives in the face of challenges. These challenges act as nurturing grounds for our resilience—an essential trait that empowers us to withstand tempests and emerge even more formidable. As we triumph over adversities, we gradually tap into our inner reservoirs, cultivating the emotional and psychological fortitude that proves indispensable in maneuvering through forthcoming obstacles.

Learning Through Experience: Wisdom in Struggles

In every challenge lies the chance to acquire wisdom through lived experiences. Emotional struggles act as mirrors, offering glimpses into the landscape of our inner selves. They beckon us to scrutinize our reactions, convictions, and methods of coping. Through the analysis of our responses to adversity, we extract valuable insights into our cognitive patterns and behavioral inclinations. This heightened self-awareness serves as the bedrock for self-enhancement and individual advancement.

Transformational Mindset: Cultivating Growth

Nurturing a mindset of transformation is a vital key to unlocking the latent potential within challenges. This mindset shift entails moving from a position of passive victimhood to one of dynamic involvement. By embracing the metamorphic potency of challenges, we cultivate a perspective that regards setbacks as pivotal markers on the path to achievement. This perspective propels us to confront difficulties with a sense of inquisitiveness, tenacity, and an enthusiasm for learning.

Embracing Challenges: The Path to Transformation

Within the intricate masterpiece of life, challenges serve as the threads that intricately weave the fabric of growth and transformation. Instead of obstructing our journey, they extend an invitation to embark on a voyage of self-discovery and evolution. Embracing these challenges bestows upon us the authority to rewrite our narratives, transforming chapters of adversity into sagas of victory. Amid these challenges, as we navigate emotional struggles, we seize the ability to craft a version of ourselves that is fortified, enlightened, and remarkably resilient. It's crucial to remember that challenges don't merely assess our strength; they also beckon us to plumb the depths of our potential, inviting us to rise to new heights.

Shifting Perspectives: From Victimhood to Empowerment

Confronted by emotional struggles, it's a common path to unwittingly tread into the territory of victimhood, succumbing to feelings of powerlessness and being engulfed by circumstances. Yet, the art of embracing challenges necessitates a shift in perspective. Rather than perceiving oneself as a victim, it's about adopting an empowered posture – one that acknowledges the hardship while simultaneously acknowledging the avenue for growth.

Cultivating Resilience: Strength Through Adversity

Resilience is the remarkable aptitude to rebound from adversity and flourish even amidst challenges. The art of converting emotional struggles into milestones demands the cultivation and nurturing of resilience. Every challenge, when met with the appropriate mindset, holds the potential to fortify this precious trait. Triumphing over emotional obstacles constructs an internal fortitude, arming us to confront forthcoming trials with enhanced composure.

Learning and Adaptation: Gaining Wisdom from Experience

Challenges frequently arrive with invaluable lessons in tow. When we open ourselves to embracing these lessons, we embark on a journey of self-discovery, uncovering insights about our strengths and areas primed for growth. Emotional struggles serve as illuminating mirrors, reflecting our thought processes, responses, and coping strategies. Through introspection and contemplation, we're equipped to pinpoint aspects necessitating enhancement and initiate purposeful endeavors to adjust and flourish.

Fostering Growth Mindset: Embracing Change

Embracing challenges nurtures a growth mindset – a conviction that capabilities and intellect can flourish through dedication and education. This mindset empowers us to perceive setbacks as chances for advancement and enhancement. By shifting our outlook, we approach emotional struggles with inquisitiveness and a readiness to delve into novel viewpoints and coping mechanisms, fostering an environment conducive to learning and progress.

Seeking Support: Connecting and Sharing

Turning emotional struggles into opportunities for growth often requires reaching out for support. Sharing our challenges with those we trust – be it friends, family, or professionals – can offer validation, direction, and a sense of belonging. These connections can assist us in navigating through difficulties, offering the motivation and reassurance necessary to continue progressing on our journey.

The Journey Toward Greater Well-Being

Embracing challenges as opportunities for growth is an ongoing voyage toward enhanced well-being. It entails recognizing that emotional struggles are inherent in life and can play a role in our personal development. Remember, it's not about evading challenges, but rather about embracing them with bravery and receptiveness, understanding that they hold the potential to guide us toward greater well-being and a more profound understanding of ourselves.

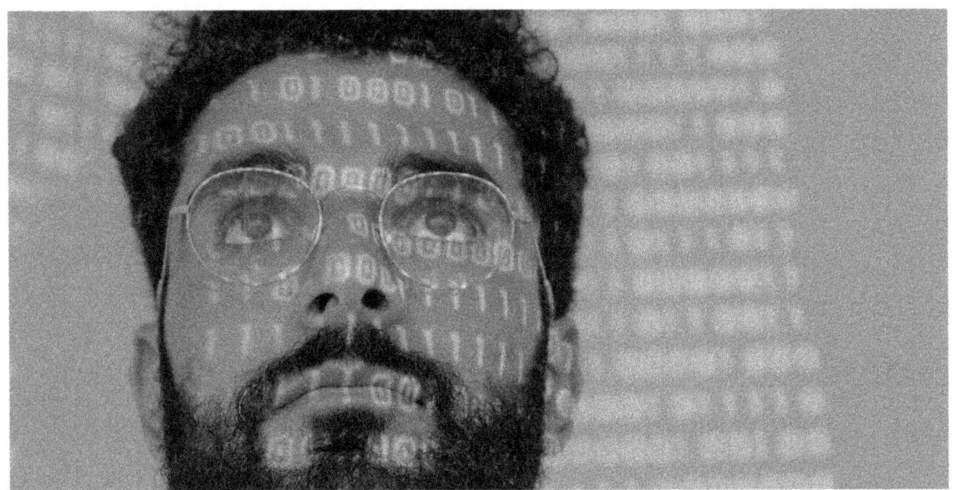

CULTIVATING EMOTIONAL INTELLIGENCE

CHAPTER 3

Exploring Emotional Intelligence: Navigating the Complex Landscape

Welcome to the journey of exploring emotional intelligence—a voyage that promises self-discovery and the enrichment of relationships. As we set sail through the dimensions of emotional intelligence, we're embarking on a quest to equip ourselves with the tools to navigate the intricate world of emotions with finesse and insight.

The Foundation: Self-Awareness

Let's start by delving into the bedrock of emotional intelligence—self-awareness. This is where our expedition truly begins. Picture it as the process of unveiling layers within ourselves, like peeling back the petals of a flower to reveal its essence. Through relatable anecdotes and examples, we'll journey through the landscape of recognizing and comprehending our own emotions. This quest for self-awareness is the compass that guides us in this expedition.

Harmonizing Emotions: Self-Regulation

Emotions are much like the currents of a river—sometimes calm and steady, and other times turbulent and unpredictable. Here, we'll explore the art of self-regulation, a skill akin to steering a ship through varying tides. By understanding how to manage and channel emotions, we gain a sense of control over our reactions and behaviors. It's about embracing the ebb and flow of our emotional waters and sailing through them with poise.

The Bridge of Connection: Empathy

In a world that often emphasizes individualism, empathy emerges as a vital bridge connecting hearts. Imagine it as walking in another person's shoes, feeling their experiences, and understanding their emotions. Through stories that resonate, we'll dive into the profound impact of empathy on relationships. It's about forging connections that go beyond surface interactions, enriching our bonds through genuine understanding.

Dance of Understanding: Effective Communication

Communication is like a dance—each word, tone, and gesture holds meaning. Here, we'll explore effective communication as a key to enhancing emotional intelligence. It's about expressing ourselves authentically while fostering understanding in others. Through this dance, we create conversations that resonate deeply, fostering connections built on emotional insight and authenticity.

From Insight to Practice: Applying Emotional Intelligence

Knowledge becomes transformative when applied. In this segment, we'll bridge theory and practice by integrating emotional intelligence into our daily lives. Through mindful practices, introspective exercises, and real-life scenarios, we'll shape our emotional intelligence. This integration creates a ripple effect, elevating our well-being and elevating the quality of our relationships.

The Journey Unfolds: Enrichment through Emotional Intelligence.

As we traverse the dimensions of emotional intelligence, we're on a journey of self-discovery and relational enrichment. These threads of emotional insight, when woven into the fabric of our lives, form the foundation of Emotional Orgasm. This mastery isn't just about personal growth; it's about nurturing harmonious connections and experiencing meaningful growth. By cultivating self-awareness, self-regulation, empathy, and effective communication, we set the stage for a life enriched by understanding and deep connections. It's an expedition that transforms us from observers to participants, shaping a future illuminated by emotional intelligence and profound relationships.

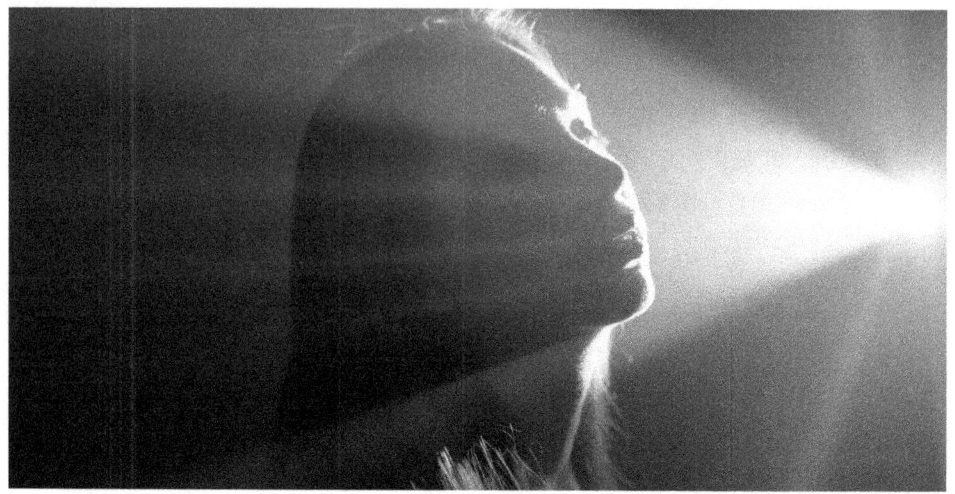

UNLEASHING THE POTENTIAL OF MINDFULNESS

CHAPTER 4

Let us dive into a chapter that unveils the remarkable power of mindfulness—a tool that holds immense promise on our journey toward Emotional Orgasm. Join me as we traverse the landscape of mindfulness, uncovering its art and learning how it can be a guiding light to cultivate present-moment awareness and detachment from distressing thoughts. Together, we'll delve into the transformative techniques, such as meditation and deep breathing, that anchor us in the present, diminish stress, and nurture emotional resilience.

Discovering Sanctuary in the Present Moment

Let us embark on a journey into the heart of mindfulness—a journey that reveals it to be more than just a trendy buzzword. It's a sanctuary, a refuge in the embrace of the present moment. With each turn of the page, I invite you to pause, redirect your focus, and immerse yourself in the serenity of now. Through relatable anecdotes, you'll come to grasp how mindfulness offers solace from the ceaseless whirlwind of thoughts, providing a haven to detach from distressing emotions and find a sense of inner calm.

Cultivating the Art of Present-Moment Awareness

In a world brimming with distractions, the art of cultivating present-moment awareness is a treasure waiting to be discovered. Allow me to guide you through the process of attuning yourself to the symphony of your surroundings, emotions, and bodily sensations. Imagine the liberation that comes with truly embracing the present, unburdened by the weight of past regrets or the uncertainties of the future. As we journey together, you'll uncover the ability to cherish the richness of each experience, paving the path for a life filled with fulfillment and authenticity.

Detachment and Non-Judgment: Keys to Navigating Life's Waves

At the heart of mindfulness lies the profound practice of detachment from judgments. As we delve into this cornerstone, you'll witness how the art of non-judgmental observation can free you from the grip of your own thoughts and emotions. It's not about stifling these emotions; instead, it's an empowering avenue toward emotional resilience. You'll learn to acknowledge your emotions, letting them flow without being engulfed by their intensity.

Anchoring in Tranquility through Mindfulness Practices

Turn the pages further, and a treasure trove of mindfulness practices unfolds before you—a collection of techniques that can anchor you in serenity. Join me in discovering the world of mindfulness meditation, a practice that nurtures focused awareness on the present. We'll also explore the art of deep breathing exercises, which become your companions amidst the chaos of daily life. These practices offer you the means to regulate your emotions, finding a sense of tranquility and a deeper connection with your inner self.

Stress Alleviation and the Harmony of Emotional Well-Being

The art of mindfulness is a potent remedy for the stress that life often presents. As I elaborate, you'll learn how centering your attention on the present moment can gradually release stress's hold on your life. Through mindfulness, you'll uncover a space—a moment to pause and choose your response, rather than reacting impulsively. Let's journey together to understand the practical applications of mindfulness, and how it can reduce stress and foster emotional well-being.

From Practice to Embodied Transformation

But our journey doesn't halt at the realm of practice; it extends into the realm of integration. I invite you to explore the idea that mindfulness isn't confined to meditation sessions—it's a philosophy that can infuse every facet of your life. Discover how to infuse mindfulness into your daily routines, turning mundane moments into opportunities for mindful presence and heightened awareness. By embracing this practice, you'll set the stage for a life marked by emotional balance, increased presence, and heightened well-being.

A Pathway to Mastery: Navigating Life with Mindfulness

As our exploration of mindfulness draws to a close, I trust you've grasped its role as a formidable tool for Emotional Orgasm. Let my guidance inspire you to embrace the present moment, detach from distressing thoughts, and navigate life's challenges with grace. Through mindfulness, you become the architect of your emotional journey—cultivating resilience, serenity, and the profound art of fully living in each moment. By practicing mindfulness, you'll discover an oasis of calm amid life's tumult, a sanctuary where Emotional Orgasm and inner peace converge. Thank you for embarking on this transformative journey of mindfulness with me.

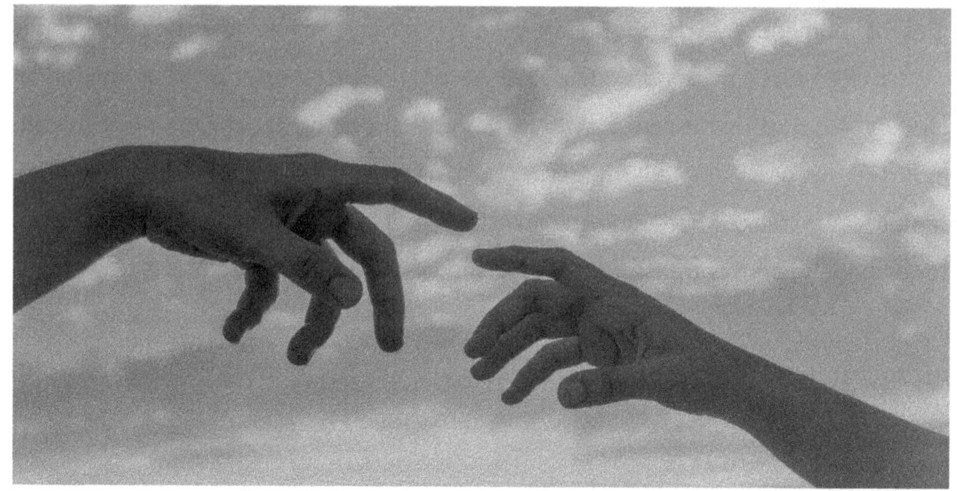

CULTIVATING MEANINGFUL BONDS

CHAPTER 5

We will now delve into the heart of nurturing meaningful relationships—a cornerstone of our emotional landscape. Join me as we navigate the intricate dynamics of connections, and uncover insights into effective communication, conflict resolution, and the art of building emotional bonds. Together, we'll equip ourselves with the tools to navigate the beautiful complexities of relationships, forging emotional connections that contribute to our overall wellness and resilience.

Foundations of Authentic Connection

At the core of every meaningful relationship lies the bedrock of authentic connection. Let's journey together as I guide you through what it truly means to connect with others on a profound level. By embracing empathy, active listening, and mutual understanding, you'll embark on a transformational journey that transcends surface interactions, creating bonds that resonate on a deeper, more meaningful frequency.

Communication: The Bridge to Genuine Understanding

Communication serves as the heartbeat of relationships, and effective communication is the bridge that leads to genuine understanding. Join me as we explore the nuances of communication, shining a light on the power of active listening, the subtlety of non-verbal cues, and the magic of empathetic expression. Through mastering the art of communication, you'll construct bridges that nurture emotional intimacy, weaving a tapestry of connections that foster authentic bonds.

Resolving Conflicts: Navigating Pathways to Growth

In the realm of relationships, conflicts are not adversaries; they are invitations to growth. Let's journey into the realm of conflict resolution, where I empower you with strategies to navigate disagreements with grace and respect. Through the art of assertive communication, addressing misunderstandings, and embracing compromise, you'll discover how conflicts can be transformed into stepping stones toward deeper understanding and emotional harmony.

Emotional Bonds: The Essence of Connection

Emotional connections are the very threads that weave relationships into a tapestry of closeness and belonging. Let me illuminate the significance of vulnerability, authenticity, and shared experiences in nurturing these bonds. Through relatable stories, you'll glimpse the enchantment of nurturing emotional intimacy—an arena where emotions are not only expressed but also deeply understood. It's within this sacred space that relationships gather strength, poised to withstand the trials that time may bring.

Cultivating Resilient Connections: The Pathway to Wellness

Nurturing meaningful relationships isn't just about forging emotional connections; it's about elevating overall well-being. Join me as I discuss how resilient relationships offer a haven in times of challenge. By nurturing open communication, mutual respect, and shared values, you'll cultivate relationships that contribute not only to your emotional health but also to your emotional resilience.

From Reflection to Transformation: Nurturing Artistry

As we journey through this chapter, remember that insights are just the beginning—transformation comes through application. Reflect on your communication patterns, your approaches to conflict, and the strength of your emotional bonds. Through guided exercises, you'll weave these insights into the fabric of your relationships, transforming them into sources of joy, support, and emotional fulfillment.

A Tapestry of Bonds: A Resilient Path

As you progress through this chapter, you're crafting a beautiful tapestry of connections that enrich your life and fortify your emotional resilience. My guidance is your compass as you navigate the intricate pathways of meaningful relationships. Remember, fostering emotional connections isn't merely an aspect of life—it's a profound investment in your personal well-being. As you embrace the lessons of effective communication, conflict resolution, and emotional bonding, you're nurturing relationships that stand as pillars of strength, enhancing your life with profound emotional connections, and guiding you on a journey of holistic well-being. Thank you for embarking on this transformative journey with me.

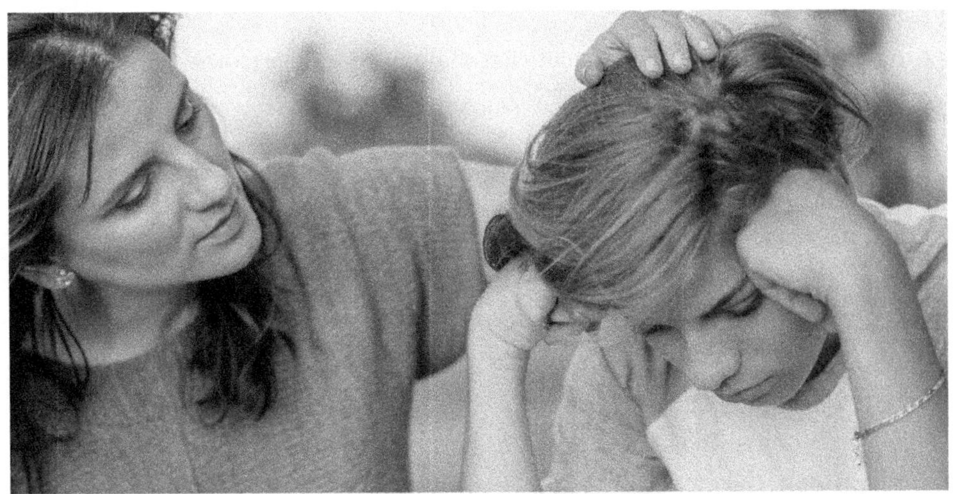

EMBRACING EMOTIONAL VULNERABILITY

CHAPTER 6

Within the tapestry of human emotions, vulnerability often stands as a misunderstood thread. In this chapter, I invite you to challenge preconceived notions, as I illuminate the strength inherent in embracing your emotional vulnerability. Together, we will journey through the depths of your emotional landscape, fostering authenticity and self-acceptance that lay the groundwork for profound healing, growth, and a more enriched emotional well-being.

The Paradox of Vulnerability: Strength in Openness

Unraveling the enigma of vulnerability, we find a paradox: the act of unveiling your emotions is not a display of fragility but a showcase of inner strength. Through relatable anecdotes and illuminating insights, you'll come to recognize that vulnerability isn't an act of submission but rather an opportunity to forge deep connections with both yourself and others.

Confronting Emotional Shadows: Unearthing Authenticity

At the core of embracing vulnerability lies the transformative journey of confronting your emotional shadows. With my guidance, you will navigate the process of acknowledging and addressing the unresolved emotional wounds that reside within. By facing the pain of your past, you will peel away layers of pretense, revealing the authentic self that exists beneath the protective veneer.

Fostering Self-Acceptance: The Key to Healing

The journey toward vulnerability leads to a remarkable discovery – the jewel of self-acceptance. Together, we will explore how embracing your imperfections and vulnerabilities is a vital step toward unconditional self-love. Through this exploration, you will come to understand that self-acceptance isn't tethered to perfection; rather, it thrives in your willingness to embrace the entirety of your emotional landscape.

The Power of Healing: Transforming Wounds into Wisdom

Embracing emotional vulnerability isn't a mere exercise in unveiling your innermost thoughts; it's a path that leads to profound healing. I will share with you the transformative potential that arises from confronting your emotional wounds head-on. By making room for grief, pain, and uncertainty, you will create a sanctuary for healing, growth, and the emergence of newfound emotional resilience.

Cultivating Emotional Well-Being: The Vulnerable Path

In the realm of emotional well-being, vulnerability emerges as a steadfast ally. Together, we will explore how embracing your emotional vulnerability can lead to heightened awareness and regulation of your emotions. By authentically acknowledging and expressing your feelings, you will cultivate healthier coping mechanisms, ultimately paving the way for an enhanced sense of overall well-being.

From Resistance to Liberation: The Journey of Vulnerability

As you delve into the heart of this chapter, you embark on a transformative journey. Guided by my insights, you will empower yourself to dismantle the barriers that have concealed your emotional vulnerability. Through introspective exercises and guided self-exploration, you will take bold steps toward liberating yourself from the weight of emotional pretense.

A Tapestry of Wholeness: Embracing Vulnerability

Within these pages, readers are weavers, threading vulnerability into the fabric of their existence. Together, we create a mosaic woven with authenticity and healing. My wisdom encourages you to discard the misconception that vulnerability equates to fragility. Instead, you will emerge with a profound realization that embracing your emotional vulnerability is a testament to your strength, a stride toward self-revelation, and a transformative odyssey that guides you to a life illuminated by authenticity, self-acceptance, and emotional well-being.

THE JOURNEY TO SELF-COMPASSION

CHAPTER 7

Within the realm of Emotional Orgasm, a transformative practice emerges—one that lays the foundation for a profound shift in how we relate to ourselves. In this chapter, I invite you to journey with me into the realm of self-compassion. Together, we will explore the intricate threads of self-kindness, mindfulness, and shared humanity, all of which weave into a tapestry of emotional resilience and inner strength.

Unveiling Self-Compassion: A Paradigm Shift

The concept of self-compassion is not a mere abstraction; it's a paradigm shift that reshapes the very fabric of our self-relationship. I will guide you through the essence of self-compassion, urging you to cast aside the cloak of self-criticism and instead embrace the embrace of self-kindness. Through relatable anecdotes, you'll come to realize the transformative power of treating yourself with the same care and empathy you would offer to your dearest friend.

Cultivating Self-Kindness: Nurturing Inner Warmth

At the heart of self-compassion lies the art of self-kindness. Together, we will delve into the practice of nurturing yourself with gentle care, particularly in moments of struggle or self-doubt. By cultivating a compassionate inner dialogue, you'll develop an emotional sanctuary that provides sustenance through the challenges of life.

Mindfulness: The Bridge to Self-Awareness

Mindfulness becomes the bridge that connects self-compassion to self-awareness. I will illustrate how the practice of mindfulness enables you to acknowledge your thoughts and emotions without judgment, paving the way for deeper self-understanding. Through mindfulness, you'll learn to cradle your experiences with open-hearted awareness, nurturing self-compassion even in the face of adversity.

Common Humanity: The Bond of Shared Experience

In the voyage toward self-compassion, the concept of common humanity serves as a unifying thread. I will guide you to recognize that your struggles are not isolated; they are part of the human experience. This realization fosters a sense of connection, inspiring you to extend to yourself the same understanding and compassion you extend to others.

The Power of Emotional Resilience: Nurturing Inner Strength

Self-compassion transcends gentleness; it's also a potent tool for cultivating emotional resilience. We will explore how self-compassion equips you to navigate life's trials with a steadier spirit. By nurturing self-kindness, mindfulness, and shared humanity, you will forge an unyielding inner strength that anchors you through life's ebbs and flows.

From Practice to Lifestyle: The Legacy of Self-Compassion

Together, we transcend the practice of self-compassion, ushering it into the realm of lifestyle. Self-compassion isn't fleeting; it's a daily commitment that reshapes your self-narrative. Through practical exercises and guided introspection, you'll integrate self-compassion into your daily routines, cultivating an emotional reservoir that sustains you through life's complexities.

A Tapestry of Self-Care: The Gift of Self-Compassion

As you traverse this chapter, you weave a tapestry interwoven with self-care, compassion, and emotional resilience. My insights empower you to embrace self-compassion as a transformative journey that nurtures your emotional well-being. Through the practice of self-kindness, mindfulness, and the recognition of shared humanity, you'll cultivate a profound inner strength, fostering a relationship with yourself characterized by empathy, warmth, and unwavering support. Within the embrace of self-compassion, you'll unearth a pathway to Emotional Orgasm—a journey that leads to a life enriched by self-love and profound inner resilience.

FROM EMOTIONAL AWARENESS TO MASTERY

CHAPTER 8

The culmination of the journey toward Emotional Orgasm comes in the form of integrating the practices and insights explored throughout this book. I invite you to join me in understanding the significance of consistent effort, self-reflection, and the embracing of setbacks as stepping stones toward learning. By embodying the principles of Emotional Orgasm, you will embark on a lifelong voyage toward nurturing resilience, fostering well-being, and experiencing a profound sense of emotional equilibrium.

The Convergence of Insights: Weaving the Tapestry

The journey to Emotional Orgasm is not a linear progression; rather, it's a tapestry meticulously woven from the threads of self-awareness, mindfulness, vulnerability, and self-compassion. I'm here to guide you in bringing these threads together, crafting a harmonious blend that empowers you to navigate life's intricacies with wisdom and grace.

Consistent Effort: Nurturing Emotional Growth

I emphasize the essential role of consistent effort in the pursuit of Emotional Orgasm. It's a reminder to approach your journey with patience and dedicated commitment. By nurturing your emotional growth through daily practices, reflective exercises, and ongoing learning, you ensure that your progress is both steadfast and sustainable.

The Art of Self-Reflection: Illuminating Insights

Self-reflection is akin to a lantern that illuminates the path toward Emotional Orgasm. I encourage you to make regular introspection a habit, examining your thoughts, emotions, and responses. Through this practice, you'll unearth valuable insights into your patterns, triggers, and overall progress, creating a space for intentional growth and evolution.

Setbacks as Stepping Stones: Lessons in Resilience

Let's reframe setbacks as stepping stones, not detours, on your journey to Emotional Orgasm. I guide you to perceive challenges as opportunities for learning and growth. By embracing these setbacks and extracting the wisdom they harbor, you will transform stumbling blocks into catalysts that propel you forward.

Embodying Mastery: A Lifelong Journey

Emotional Orgasm isn't a destination to reach; it's a lifelong expedition of growth and refinement. I'll show you how to embody the principles you've acquired, weaving them seamlessly into your daily existence. By applying the practices of emotional awareness, self-compassion, and vulnerability, you'll lay a firm foundation that supports you through every twist and turn.

The Ripple Effect: Radiating Well-Being

As you embrace Emotional Orgasm, you become an agent of positive change. I emphasize how the well-being you cultivate through this journey extends beyond yourself. By embodying emotional balance and resilience, you inspire others and create a ripple effect of well-being that extends through your relationships, communities, and beyond.

The Legacy of Mastery: A Life of Fulfillment

In this final chapter, you'll grasp the profound legacy that your journey toward Emotional Orgasm is forming. My guidance encourages you to approach life with a newfound sense of emotional equilibrium and wisdom. By internalizing the principles of consistent effort, self-reflection, and resilience, you embark on a path that transcends the pages of this book, leading you toward a life of fulfillment, enriched relationships, and a profound connection with your own emotional landscape.

The Masterpiece Unveiled: A Life Well-Lived

In this chapter, we add the finishing strokes to your emotional masterpiece. With my guidance, you step into the realm of Emotional Orgasm, equipped with insights, practices, and a deep understanding of yourself. By embracing the journey, you unveil a life well-lived—a life characterized by resilience, well-being, and an unwavering sense of emotional balance. As you continue to paint the canvas of your emotions, you transform into the architect of your emotional landscape, creating a legacy resonating with authenticity, growth, and lasting fulfillment.

CONCLUSION

"Dance with the Shadow: Emotions Unveiled" by Dr. Vivek S. Ph.D. Ph.D., iGCBT, serves as a comprehensive guide that empowers readers to embark on a transformative journey toward Emotional Orgasm. Through a harmonious blend of evidence-based strategies, relatable anecdotes, and compassionate guidance, I provide individuals with the essential tools to navigate life's challenges, enhance emotional intelligence, and foster enduring well-being. This book stands not just as a roadmap to emotional resilience, but also extends an invitation to embark on a lifelong exploration of the intricate landscape of emotions. As you delve into the wisdom within these pages, you'll find yourself on a profound path of self-discovery, empowerment, and emotional transformation.

www.ingramcontent.com/pod-product-compliance
Lightning Source LLC
Chambersburg PA
CBHW070815280726
48660CB00015B/967